MW01105112

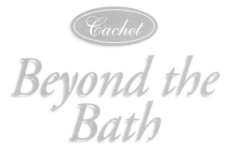

Beyond the Bath

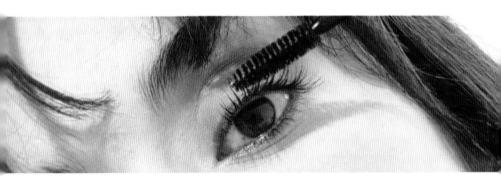

TOP THAT!

Copyright © 2004 Top That! Publishing Inc,
25031 W. Avenue Stanford,
Suite #60, Valencia, CA 91355
All rights reserved
www.topthatpublishing.com

contents

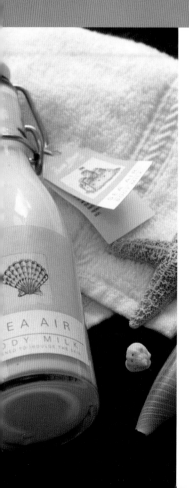

Ready to celebrate the simplicity of feeling healthy and looking good? Then read on.

This book is all about enhancing your beauty routines and makeup techniques, including advice on how to manage stress and exercise tips. With emphasis on simplicity, *Beyond the Bath* takes a healthy, natural approach to mind and body maintenance—while still acknowledging the joy of finding the ideal lipstick, and how the perfect haircut can really make you feel great.

Lifestyle!

Your beauty regime will, no doubt, depend on your lifestyle—but it need not require excessive time, money or hassle. The beauty of a good regime lies in its simplicity!

The appearance and genuine health of your skin, hair, nails, and body will be a direct result of the time and effort that you have dedicated to them. For a regime to be effective it needs to be balanced in many areas, and this may involve altering your daily routine. All of the makeup you can buy will still look tired on a face that has not had enough sleep.

The way in which the body operates means that if external care, such as moisturizing your face, is not balanced with a nutritious diet, plenty of water, regular exercise, and minimal negative effects such as smoking, all of the positives will be to no avail.

Changes...

Creating a set routine will help ensure you don't neglect or forget elements of your beauty regime. However, it needs to be flexible enough to cope with things that will inevitably change, like scalp condition, oiliness of the skin, and climate. Knowledge of how to deal with many different skin and hair types will arm you for these changes.

Finally, don't feel guilty about taking time out for you. If other people rely on you, they will understand that you need time to relax, pamper, and maintain your body, and they will want you at your best.

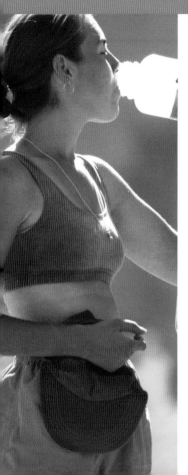

It is difficult when you are so busy to take the time out to spend even a few minutes taking care of your body—particularly when it is just something to make you feel good. Here are some quick things that you can do that will have brilliant results and give you a boost to last the rest of the day.

body of water

Ideally, you should drink between eight and ten glasses of water a day. You should not wait until you're thirsty because this means your body has already lost more water than it should have done. Water not only hydrates your body, but helps your organs function efficiently and keeps your hair silky, nails healthy, and skin radiant.

brisk walk

If you are spending all day at a desk, particularly in front of a computer, it is important to take regular breaks. A brisk ten-minute walk in your lunch hour will stretch your muscles, refocus your eyes, and relax your mind ready for work in the afternoon.

de-stress self-massage

Just a few minutes of self-massage will help relieve tension and stress. Using a little oil, place your thumbs on your temples and stretch your fingers across your forehead. Move your fingers from the center to your temples and back, in a firm, circular motion. The neck and shoulders are classic tension points. Use your hands

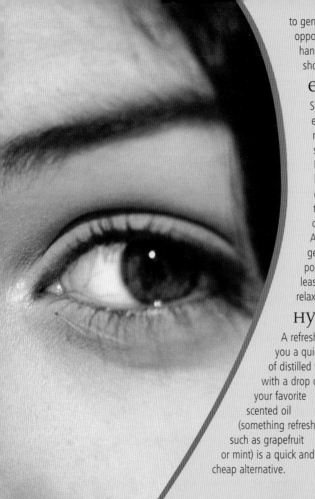

to gently squeeze and firmly massage the opposite shoulder muscles. Move your hands firmly across the top of the shoulder to the neck and back.

eye revival

Signs of weariness and stress are often evident around the eyes. Although nothing will fix this like a good night's sleep, this quick fix will perk you up! Place cucumber slices or a used tea bag (cooled and squeezed) over your eyes and lie back for ten minutes. The tea bag will firm the skin, while the cucumber is cooling and refreshing. Alternatively, there are a number of gel-filled eye masks available. Simply pop them into the refrigerator for at least thirty minutes, then sit back and relax with the mask covering your eyes.

hydrating spray

A refreshing spritz from an atomizer can give you a quick lift. A spray bottle of distilled water with a drop of your favorite scented oil (something refreshing such as grapefruit or mint) is a quick and cheap alternative.

5

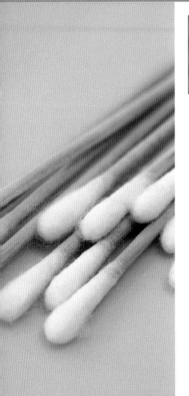

It is surprising how few tools we actually need to apply beauty and makeup products, but amazing how many gadgets we can accumulate. There are a number of tools, however, that you really will, or already do, use every day.

Beauty Basics

Keep your tools clean. Wash your brushes and sponges at least once a week. Use a mild soap detergent, or facial cleanser under running water, then allow them to air-dry thoroughly.

Cotton balls—Ideal for many jobs such as applying cleanser and removing makeup.

Cotton swabs—Handy for applying small amounts of foundation or for neatening up mascara, eyeliner, and lipstick.

Tweezers—Choose good tweezers with a lot of spring-back and a slanted edge to pluck hairs.

Emery boards and cuticle sticks—An essential part of every manicure kit.

Sponges—Foundation applied with a sponge looks soft and sheer.

Pencil sharpener—Keep your eyebrow, eyeliner, and lipliner pencils sharpened. You'll need two or three sizes of sharpeners to match your collection of pencils.

Eyelash curler—Use before applying mascara to widen the appearance of the eyes. Curling lashes after you apply mascara can cause lashes to break. Ensure the curler has foam padding to protect the lashes.

BRUSHES

Different brushes can help an amateur master techniques like a professional.

Powder brush—The largest brush in your collection fluffs finishing powder onto your face, softens foundation, or blends blusher.

Blusher brush—Fluffy blusher brushes, cut on an angle, fit comfortably over the cheekbone. Brushes in blush compacts are usually too small and pick up too much color.

Eyeliner brush—Use this narrow, domed brush to line the eyes with eyeshadow, or to smudge eyeliner.

Eyeshadow brushes—There are a number of types available. A soft, fluffy brush is ideal to wash color over the whole lid; and a small, soft, slanted brush will apply contour color into the crease under the socket bone.

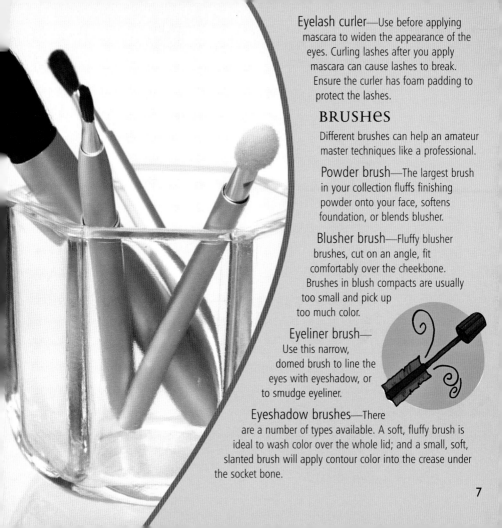

7

the Body in and out of the Bath

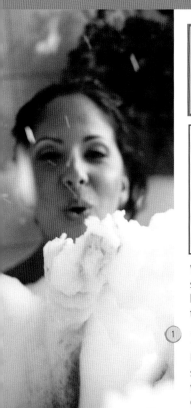

No matter what sins you may have committed against your skin in the past, it is never too late to start taking care of it. You don't need to go out and buy every product on the shelves—there are lots of treatments that you can make with ingredients from your kitchen!

⚠ WARNING

Essential oils enter the bloodstream through the skin. NEVER apply them directly to your skin as they can be extremely potent. Dilute in a carrier oil and ALWAYS do a patch test first.

Patch test: Mix one drop of the essential oil into a teaspoon of carrier oil. Rub a little of the mixture on the inside of your wrist. Leave uncovered and unwashed for 24 hours. If experience no irritation the oil is safe to use in a diluted form.

Whether you love a refreshing, cold shower, or a long, relaxing soak with bath salts, there is lots of fun to be had, with lots of lotions and potions that can help your skin look taut, tanned, and terrific. Follow the easy steps for a great body care regime.

① before you get into the tub

Before you get into the bath, use a body brush in long, sweeping strokes over the body. Start at the feet and move up the legs, working towards the heart. Dry-skin brushing will stimulate circulation and improve lymphatic drainage.

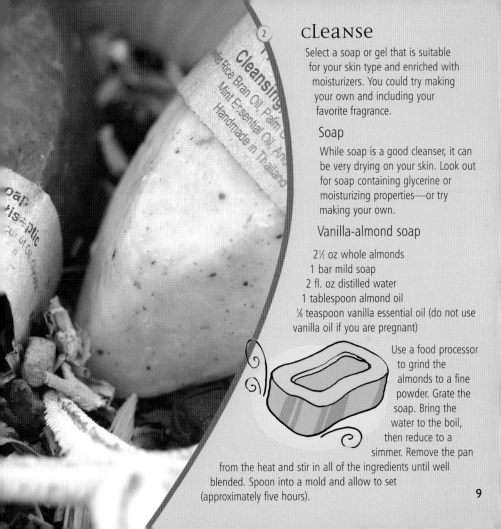

cLeanse

Select a soap or gel that is suitable for your skin type and enriched with moisturizers. You could try making your own and including your favorite fragrance.

Soap

While soap is a good cleanser, it can be very drying on your skin. Look out for soap containing glycerine or moisturizing properties—or try making your own.

Vanilla-almond soap

2½ oz whole almonds
1 bar mild soap
2 fl. oz distilled water
1 tablespoon almond oil
⅛ teaspoon vanilla essential oil (do not use vanilla oil if you are pregnant)

Use a food processor to grind the almonds to a fine powder. Grate the soap. Bring the water to the boil, then reduce to a simmer. Remove the pan from the heat and stir in all of the ingredients until well blended. Spoon into a mold and allow to set (approximately five hours).

9

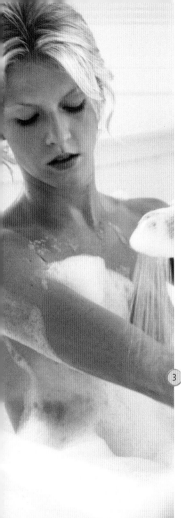

Bath bomb (makes 2-3 balls)

These fizzy balls of fun are easy to make at home and are normally infused with fragrant and therapeutic oils. They can make an ideal gift too!

9 oz baking soda (sodium bicarbonate)
2½ teaspoons citric acid (sifted or finely ground)
2½ teaspoons cornstarch
dry herbs or flowers (optional)
2½ tablespoons sweet almond oil
¾ tablespoon water
¼ teaspoon of lavender essential oil
A few drops of food coloring (optional)

Mix all the dry ingredients together. Use an old jar with a lid to mix the wet ingredients—shake well. Slowly pour the wet ingredients into the dry, and mix with your hands. The mixture needs to be damp enough to hold together. If needed, mist with witch hazel or water. Press the mixture into the molds. To make a ball, use a two-part sphere, fill each side, and then press together. Allow the bombs to dry in their mold for about three hours. Remove from the mold and dry for one week before use. Cover with tissue paper and store in a dry place.

3 exfoliate

Exfoliation improves the circulation, invigorates the skin, and gets rid of dead skin cells, making it easier for moisturizers to be absorbed. Exfoliate the entire body at least once or twice a week using loofahs, washcloths, silk mitts, or body scrubs.

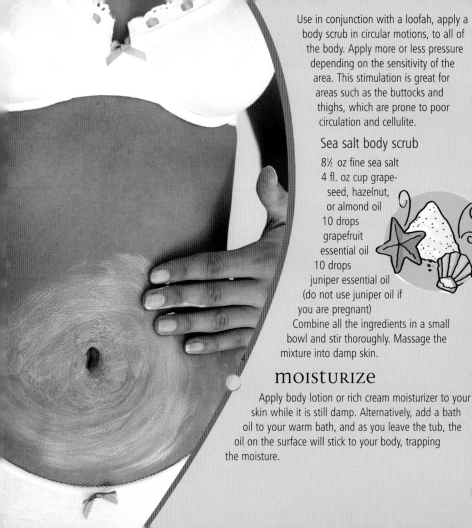

Use in conjunction with a loofah, apply a body scrub in circular motions, to all of the body. Apply more or less pressure depending on the sensitivity of the area. This stimulation is great for areas such as the buttocks and thighs, which are prone to poor circulation and cellulite.

Sea salt body scrub

8½ oz fine sea salt
4 fl. oz cup grape-
  seed, hazelnut,
  or almond oil
10 drops
  grapefruit
  essential oil
10 drops
  juniper essential oil
(do not use juniper oil if
you are pregnant)
Combine all the ingredients in a small bowl and stir thoroughly. Massage the mixture into damp skin.

moisturize

Apply body lotion or rich cream moisturizer to your skin while it is still damp. Alternatively, add a bath oil to your warm bath, and as you leave the tub, the oil on the surface will stick to your body, trapping the moisture.

face care and facials

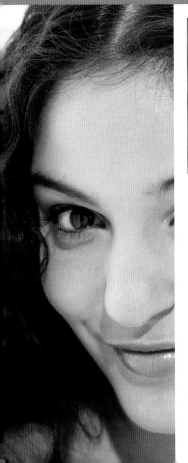

The skin on the face is different from every other part of your body, and no two people have exactly the same skin type. Your facial regime should be as individual as you are and can be as easy, or as involved, as you choose to make it. Despite what cosmetic companies may have you believe, you need very few products to maintain healthy, radiant skin. Your daily, basic skin care need only include cleansing, toning, moisturizing, and sun care. This twice-a-day routine can be enhanced with a home facial, including exfoliation, masks, and serums.

what is your skin type?

Normal—If you're lucky enough to have normal skin, just focus on maintaining that wonderful balance.

Dry—This skin type has a lack of oil and moisture in the skin.

Oily – This is characterized by its tendency to break out in spots and blemishes, with large open pores and an oily surface.

Combination—You will have a majority of normal skin, with an oily "T-zone." This T-shaped patch includes your forehead, nose, and chin.

Sensitive—Can be identified by irritations, such as blotchy red marks, or chapped skin.

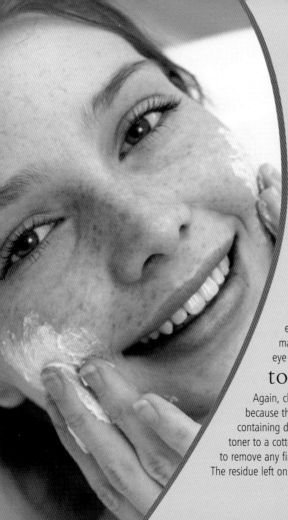

cLeansing

Cleansing is essential to remove makeup, oily residue, and impurities from the skin's surface. To ensure that the cleanser will not be too harsh, you need to select one specifically for your skin type.

Follow the manufacturer's instructions for applying and removing your cleanser. While some will mean washing your face using your cleanser and rinsing with warm water, others may only need to be applied and removed using a cotton ball. To ensure that all of the cleanser is removed from the skin, follow with a toner.

As the skin around the eyes and the eyes themselves are very sensitive, eye makeup should only be removed with an eye makeup remover.

toning

Again, choose a toner for your skin type, because they come in many different strengths, containing different levels of alcohol. Apply the toner to a cotton ball and gently wipe over the skin to remove any final traces of makeup, oil, and grime. The residue left on the cotton ball may amaze you!

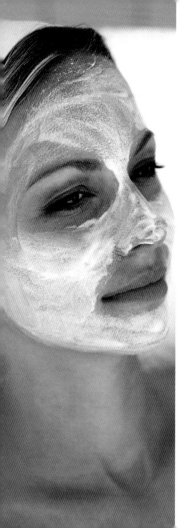

moisturizing

If you do nothing else, give your skin a hydrating lift with a moisturizer formulated for your skin. Since oil and water are not the same, even oily skin needs moisturizing. A moisturizer will provide a protective barrier and prevent the evaporation of your skin's natural moisture. Rehydrating your skin can also help minimize the appearance of fine lines.

Dot a small amount of moisturizer onto the cheeks, chin, and forehead and blend gently in an upward motion, remembering to moisturize the neck as well. Keep the movements gentle—there's no need to tug or pull the skin. Be careful not to apply to the eye area (unless your product is recommended for this area) because additional moisture can cause puffiness.

Night creams contain more nutrients that help increase the skin's ability to retain moisture. Your makeup will not sit well on a night cream so save this product for just before bed.

sun care

UVA and UVB rays from the sun can be harmful to the skin, causing dehydration, loss of elasticity, and an increased risk of skin cancer. Use a daily moisturizer containing a sunscreen to protect the skin from the sun's harmful rays.

exfoliating

A gentle exfoliant will clear the skin of impurities and dead skin cells, and give you a fresh, clear canvas ready to absorb your moisturizer. Exfoliants can be used from once a day to weekly depending on the abrasiveness of the product. Depending on your type of product, you can do this either before, or instead of, cleansing.

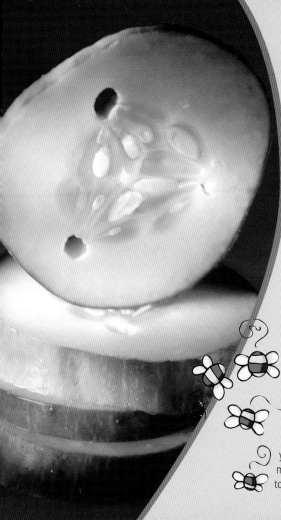

masks

While regular cleansing removes surface impurities, a facial mask will help draw them to the surface. Exfoliating masks will add extra lift and leave your skin feeling soft and smooth. Apply once a week, after cleansing, and before toning, during your normal routine.

You can also use ingredients from your kitchen to make face masks. As a general rule, cucumber and mint are natural refreshers; oats exfoliate; cream cleanses and softens; lemon juice tones and refreshes. Mix and match these ingredients, add a few other items from your cupboards and you will have cheap, accessible treatments in no time!

Honey-peach mask

1 large, skinned peach
3 teaspoons honey
2 tablespoons plain, natural yogurt

Works like magic and tastes great! Mash the ingredients until you have a workable paste. Pat evenly over your face and neck avoiding your eyes. Lie back and relax for about ten minutes. Rinse well with warm water, tone, and moisturize.

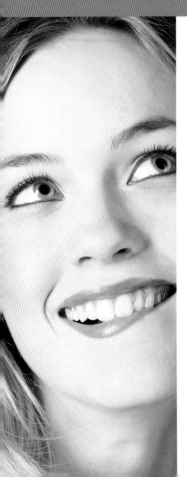

> No one will deny that makeup transforms our looks and can make us feel great. You can look radiant with natural makeup that works with your features and skin tone. And remember—less is more.

THE COLOR of YOU!

There are two basic color categories, warm, and cool. You can tell which color you are by the tone of your skin, hair, and eyes. By wearing colors that match your tone you can enhance your natural beauty.

Warm features:

Eyes—Green, blue, turquoise, golden brown, or hazel.
Skin—Pale with peach or a gold hue, brown with golden undertones, or golden tan.
Hair—Red, highlighted with red, strawberry blond, or gray with yellow tones.

Warm complexions are neither very pale or dark, and generally include all the medium skin tones such as olive, and honey tones with yellow undertones.

Best makeup colors:

Cheeks—Bronze, peach, and apricot.
Lips—Cherry, brick or yellow-reds, plums, bronze, and apricot-browns.

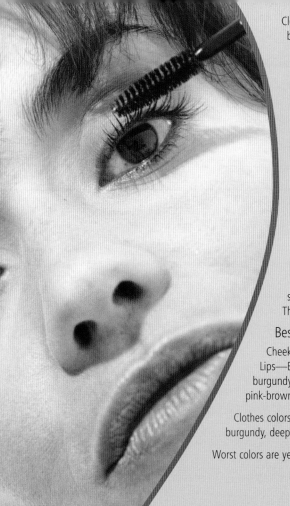

Clothes colors should be bright reds, blues, or earth tones like khaki, olive, and rust.

Worst colors are dull, pale pink, and pinkish blue.

Cool features:

Eyes—Dark blue, blue-gray, deep brown, black-brown, or hazel with blue or gray flecks.
Skin—Olive, bronze tan, chocolate brown, any skin tone with pink in the cheeks or pink undertones.
Hair—Golden blond, dark to medium brown, blue-black, or gray.

Cool complexions include extreme shades at both ends of the skin tone spectrum: pale, rosy or dark ebony. The undertone is pinkish-blue.

Best makeup colors:

Cheeks—Pink and rosy.
Lips—Blue-reds, berry, soft rose, mauve, burgundy, maroon-brown, raisin, eggplant, and pink-browns.

Clothes colors should be deep tones like navy, burgundy, deep indigo, or chalky pastels.

Worst colors are yellow and orange.

17

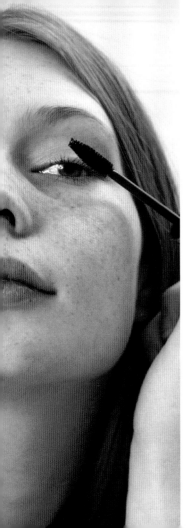

foundation and powders

It is best to keep foundation and powders as light and natural as possible, with a color close to your skin tone. When purchasing a foundation you should try to see the color in natural light to find its true shade. You also need to consider the season; for instance, if you are coming into winter your color may need to be lighter than during the summer. Thick foundation can be mixed with some light moisturizer to give a sheer finish.

Apply foundation to a clean, moisturized face. Blend evenly, and create a natural line around the jaw-line, ears, eyes, and lips. Applying powder onto the foundation will help it set and help achieve a flawless look. Foundations with ingredients that reflect light, and shimmering loose powder, make the skin look radiant.

Certain complexion problems can be helped with specific colors. Use green concealer to hide red-toned blemishes like pimples, scars, and broken capillaries. A yellow concealer will cover up dark under-eye color.

cheeks and blusher

Apply blusher sparingly and spread slightly beyond the cheek, in a diagonal, upward-sweeping motion, and blend well.

eyelids, brows and lashes

Draw, or powder eyebrows, in the direction of the hair growth with a color matching their natural color. Applying a base color to your entire eyelid will help the shadow last all day. eyeshadow comes in various forms—powder, gel, and cream. Using various shades, from light just under the brow, to dark above the lashes, will give your eyes depth and definition.

Lining your eyes with a pencil helps shape the eyes, and open them up. A powder eyeshadow can also double as an eyeliner —wet a brush with some water and dip into the eyeshadow. Add length and thickness to lashes with volumizing mascara, but beware that some can make lashes gluggy. For day, a natural-looking waterproof mascara is ideal.

Lips and Lipsticks

Use a lipliner that is slightly lighter or close to your lipstick color. Color your lips fully with a lipliner before applying lipstick or lip gloss. This will help the color last and will give a balanced shade to the lips.

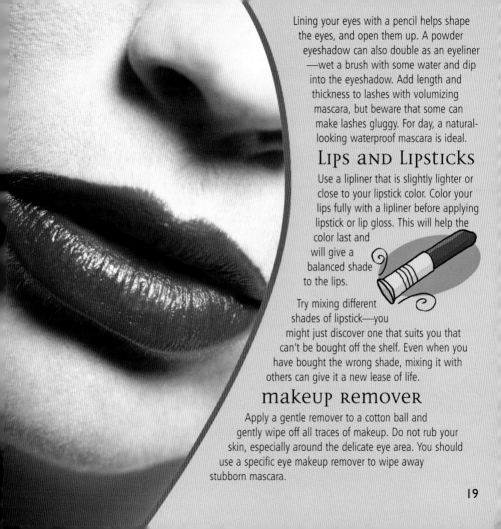

Try mixing different shades of lipstick—you might just discover one that suits you that can't be bought off the shelf. Even when you have bought the wrong shade, mixing it with others can give it a new lease of life.

makeup remover

Apply a gentle remover to a cotton ball and gently wipe off all traces of makeup. Do not rub your skin, especially around the delicate eye area. You should use a specific eye makeup remover to wipe away stubborn mascara.

perfume and fragrance

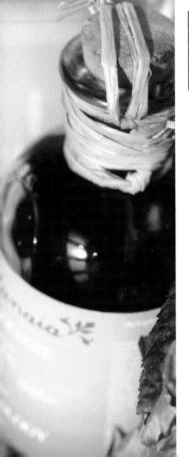

Fragrance is a very personal choice and can have a dramatic effect on your mood. A light citrus perfume will have you bounding out of the door, whereas a woody oriental can make you feel subdued and thoughtful.

which fragrance?

To relieve stress: lavender, vanilla.
Energize and uplift: citrus, green tea, grapefruit, lemon, and pine.
To feel sensual: sandalwood, musk, and jasmine.

There are three main categories of perfume—floral, oriental, and chypre; plus many other variations such as woody, musk, aquatic, spicy, and fruity. A perfume contains from ten to more than 250 ingredients which can include notes like ginger, peppercorns, vanilla, green tea, grapefruit, rose, fig leaves—the list goes on.

Each perfume is divided into three stages—beginning, middle, and end. These are the different stages of perfume evaporation. This is why a perfume will smell different when you first spray it, an hour later, and at the end of the day.

The strength and longevity of your fragrance is determined by how much perfume oil it contains. Eau de parfum, the strongest and most lasting fragrance, contains about 15-18 percent perfume oil. Eau de toilette is French for "toilet water" and is ideal for everyday use. It contains about 4-8 percent perfume oil.

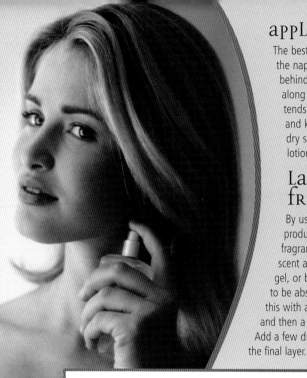

application tips

The best spots to apply perfume are the nape (back) of the neck, cleavage, behind the ears, inner elbow, and along the collar bones. Oily skin tends to retain fragrance for longer and keeps it stronger. If you have dry skin, apply an oil-based skin lotion before putting on perfume.

Layer your fragrance!

By using a number of different products with your favorite fragrance, you will trail a cloud of scent all day. Start by using a shower gel, or bath oil, to allow the fragrance to be absorbed by your skin. Follow this with an all-over body moisturizer, and then a spray of your eau de toilette. Add a few drops of perfume sparingly for the final layer.

friendly fragrance tips!

- To prolong your perfume's life, place it in a cool, dry, dark place. This will help prevent evaporation, discoloration, and alteration of the smell.

- Be careful applying perfume when wearing clothes, as it can stain delicate fabrics such as silk.

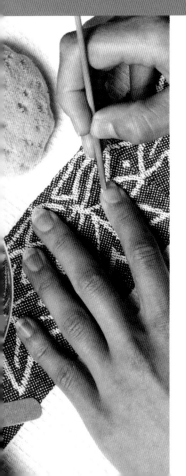

> Maintaining healthy natural nails is not as difficult as you may think. Like hair, nails are usually healthiest in their natural state, requiring just a bit of nail polish for protection, and regular applications of moisturizer.

healthy nail care tips

- Don't clip nails to shorten them. Use an emery board to file nails down to size.

- Use nail polish remover infrequently, especially if it contains acetone.

- Use rubber gloves when nails will be exposed to water or household cleaners. These will quickly dry out nails, leaving them brittle.

- Apply hand cream as often as possible.

- Do not cut the cuticle. Push it back gently with a cuticle stick or a rubber-tipped cuticle-pusher.

- Never peel or scrape off nail polish or use metal instruments on the nail surface. This will damage the protective cells of the nail.

- Frequent nail splitting can indicate dehydration. Drink more fluids and use an oil designed to penetrate the nail plate.

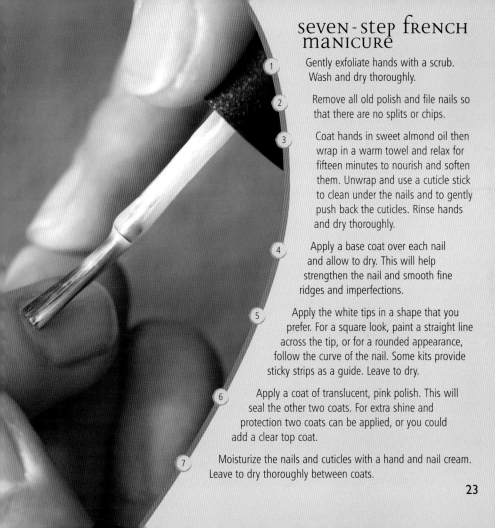

seven-step french manicure

1. Gently exfoliate hands with a scrub. Wash and dry thoroughly.

2. Remove all old polish and file nails so that there are no splits or chips.

3. Coat hands in sweet almond oil then wrap in a warm towel and relax for fifteen minutes to nourish and soften them. Unwrap and use a cuticle stick to clean under the nails and to gently push back the cuticles. Rinse hands and dry thoroughly.

4. Apply a base coat over each nail and allow to dry. This will help strengthen the nail and smooth fine ridges and imperfections.

5. Apply the white tips in a shape that you prefer. For a square look, paint a straight line across the tip, or for a rounded appearance, follow the curve of the nail. Some kits provide sticky strips as a guide. Leave to dry.

6. Apply a coat of translucent, pink polish. This will seal the other two coats. For extra shine and protection two coats can be applied, or you could add a clear top coat.

7. Moisturize the nails and cuticles with a hand and nail cream. Leave to dry thoroughly between coats.

foot care and pedicure

Your feet take a pounding! They absorb the shock and pressure from around 9,000 steps a day. If you want them to look great in summer sandals, take care of them all year round. A pedicure is quick and easy to do and will make your feet feel soft and smooth.

1. Start by removing any old nail polish.

2. Clip toenails straight across to prevent ingrown nails. File them in one direction, straight across.

3. Soak your feet in warm water to soften calluses and cuticles. Add some Epsom salts or scented bath oil. As an alternative you could try soaking them in a bowl of warm milk. Heat the milk in the microwave until warm, and comfortable to touch. Soaking you feet in the milk will gently cleanse, soften, and hydrate the skin and nails.

4. Scrub rough patches with a wet pumice stone or foot exfoliant—be gentle and don't over-scrub. You can make your own foot scrub from sea salt and lemon juice. Rub this into feet to help soften the skin, and remove discoloration.

5. Scrub your toenails with a nail brush before rinsing them in cool water.

6. While your skin is slightly damp, apply a mixture of one teaspoon of honey and one teaspoon of olive oil. Cover your feet in plastic wrap and then a pair of cotton socks for thirty minutes.

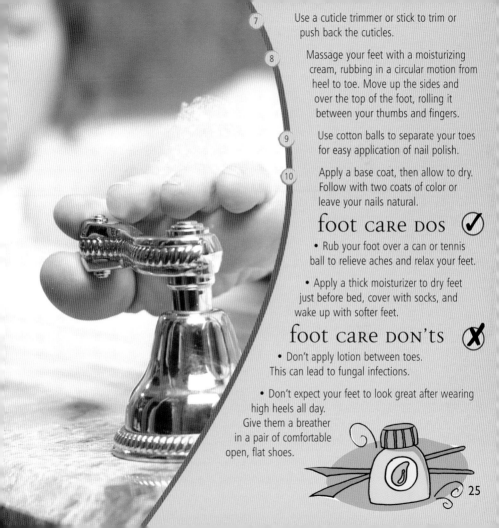

7. Use a cuticle trimmer or stick to trim or push back the cuticles.

8. Massage your feet with a moisturizing cream, rubbing in a circular motion from heel to toe. Move up the sides and over the top of the foot, rolling it between your thumbs and fingers.

9. Use cotton balls to separate your toes for easy application of nail polish.

10. Apply a base coat, then allow to dry. Follow with two coats of color or leave your nails natural.

foot care dos ✓

• Rub your foot over a can or tennis ball to relieve aches and relax your feet.

• Apply a thick moisturizer to dry feet just before bed, cover with socks, and wake up with softer feet.

foot care don'ts ✗

• Don't apply lotion between toes. This can lead to fungal infections.

• Don't expect your feet to look great after wearing high heels all day. Give them a breather in a pair of comfortable open, flat shoes.

25

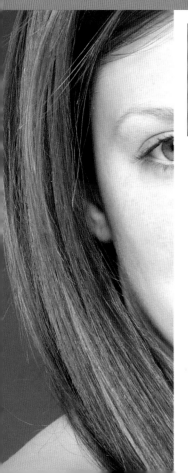

Hair care

Your hair is one of the first things that people will notice about you, and can reflect your overall health. Just like your skin and nails, it does need special attention to look its shiny, bouncy best. Your hair is such a versatile feature it can be used to achieve a totally different look—cheaply, easily and either temporarily or permanently.

a good cut

If you are considering making a dramatic change, it is always best to get advice. Ask your friends, family, and a salon professional what new look they think will suit you. Remember to consider how much time you have to dedicate to maintenance and daily styling.

coloring

A dynamic color change can really lift your spirits. Find out the difference between the different kinds of color, how long each will last, and how they will affect your hair. If you are planning on a shade lighter than your existing one, consult a professional. Make sure you consider your skin tone and eye color when making your choice.

hair extensions

This is a fun way to get a temporary new look. Most hair only grows around six inches a year, so this is a great way to shortcut nature.

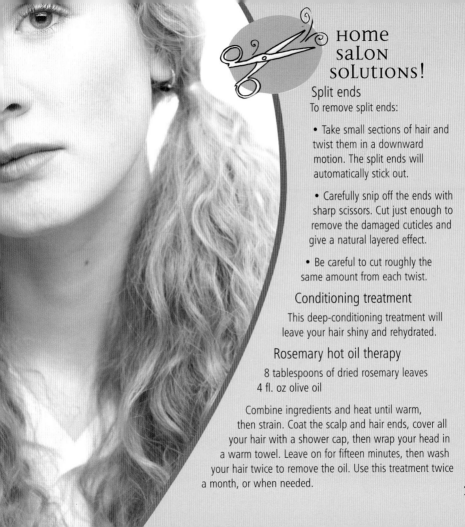

Home Salon Solutions!

Split ends

To remove split ends:

- Take small sections of hair and twist them in a downward motion. The split ends will automatically stick out.

- Carefully snip off the ends with sharp scissors. Cut just enough to remove the damaged cuticles and give a natural layered effect.

- Be careful to cut roughly the same amount from each twist.

Conditioning treatment

This deep-conditioning treatment will leave your hair shiny and rehydrated.

Rosemary hot oil therapy

8 tablespoons of dried rosemary leaves
4 fl. oz olive oil

Combine ingredients and heat until warm, then strain. Coat the scalp and hair ends, cover all your hair with a shower cap, then wrap your head in a warm towel. Leave on for fifteen minutes, then wash your hair twice to remove the oil. Use this treatment twice a month, or when needed.

27

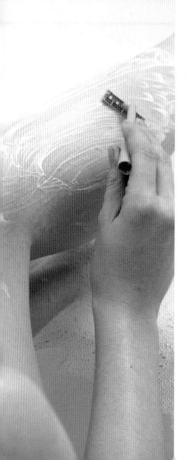

There are many different ways that you can remove unwanted hair, and thankfully, not all of them are painful. If you can't stand the thought of "pain for gain," why not look at these less traumatic alternatives.

The first thing that you need to decide is if you want to remove the hair temporarily or permanently. Temporary hair removal can be done as either depilation (removing part of the hair from above the skin) or epilation (removing the hair and its root).

Depilation methods include shaving, dissolving creams, and buffers and can last from several hours to several days. Epilation is best achieved with wax, tweezers, or rotary epilators and can last up to several weeks. Permanent removal of hair can be costly and can cause adverse effects. Different parts of the body benefit best from different hair removal methods.

temporary depilation

Shaving—Quick and easy, shaving produces instant, hassle-free results, and is suitable for most parts of the body. It is widely believed that shaving causes hair to grow back thicker and faster, but this is not true.

Creams—Fast and inexpensive, caustic creams dissolve the hair above the skin. Always do a patch test before use because the chemicals can cause skin irritation or burns.

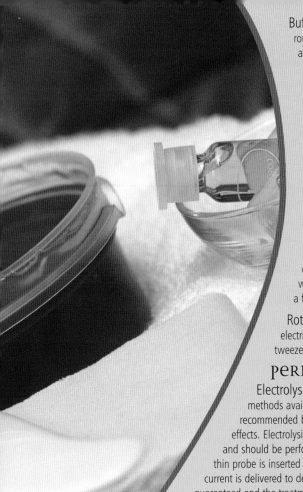

Buffers—Ideal for fine leg hair, these rough mitts or strips buff away the hair, and exfoliate the skin at the same time.

temporary epilation

Waxing—Use either hot or cold wax depending on the area of the body. Cold wax is best used for larger areas such as the legs and arms. It is applied using a spatula or roller, a fabric strip is then applied, and then pulled off quickly taking the hair and the root with it. Hot wax is a lot thicker and is ideal for smaller sensitive areas such as the bikini line, underarms, and eyebrows. It is applied directly to the area and then removed when it is thick and tacky to touch, using a fabric strip.

Rotary epilator—These look similar to an electric razor, but have rows of rotating tweezers that pull the hair out by the roots.

permanent

Electrolysis—Although there are other permanent methods available, many of these are not widely recommended because of mediocre results or side-effects. Electrolysis is widely available in beauty parlors and should be performed by a trained professional. A hair-thin probe is inserted into the hair follicle where an electric current is delivered to destroy the hair's root. Results are not guaranteed and the treatment can be expensive.

NUTRITION

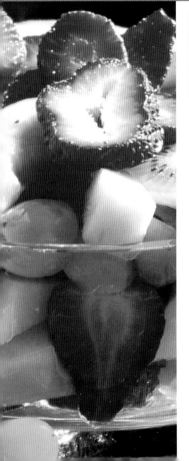

It is said that "we are what we eat," and it is true that our diet has a direct impact on every element of our body, such as the health of our skin, nails, hair, and our energy levels.

NUTRITIONAL NEEDS

Our specific nutrition and energy needs are different at various times in our lives. Although every individual is different, most adults aged from 19 to 50 should maintain a balanced diet with plenty of starchy foods, fruit, and vegetables. Only a moderate amount of meat (or its alternatives), milk and milk products, and small amounts of food and drinks containing fat and sugar, should be consumed daily.

The bodies of young children and adolescents are busy growing and developing, so they need a constant supply of energy delivered in regular, healthy snacks. It is important to instill healthy eating habits in children while they are young, because eating preferences are established early in life. As people get older, they tend to eat less. To keep energy levels up, and to ensure a constant supply of vitamins and minerals, fresh fruit and vegetables are vital.

At every stage in our lives it is vital to keep the intake of food in line with the amount of energy that we use. This will help prevent conditions like obesity, diabetes, and heart disease.

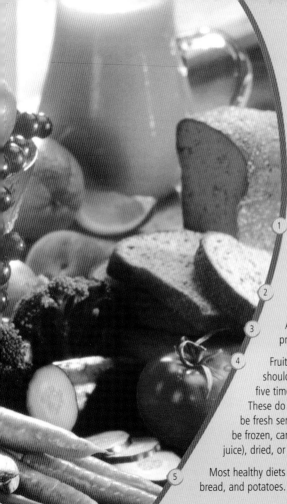

UNDERSTANDING THE FOOD PYRAMID

Always bear these golden rules in mind: balance, moderation, variation. This will ensure your diet is made up of the foods that will provide you with the nutrition needed.

Follow these guidelines for basic daily requirements:

1. Chocolate, cookies, cakes, candy, fast food, and other "treats" should be eaten rarely—once a day at the most.

2. No more than two or three servings of meat, poultry, fish, and alternatives.

3. A maximum of three portions of dairy produce such as milk, cheese, and yogurt.

4. Fruit and vegetables should be eaten three to five times a day. These do not need to be fresh servings, they can be frozen, canned (in natural juice), dried, or juiced.

5. Most healthy diets should contain cereals, rice, bread, and potatoes.

specialist diets

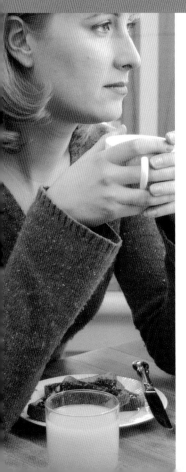

Not all diets are about losing weight—but this can be a side-effect of healthy eating and an improved lifestyle. Whether you make positive changes for 48 hours, 28 days, or a lifetime, you can still reap the rewards.

which diet?

There are loads of fad diets around, and some have more merit than others. You may find that one of these life-changing regimes will add vitality, energy, and good long-term health. Of course, you should always consult your doctor before making any dramatic alterations to your diet.

macrobiotic diet

Macrobiotics is the philosophy that encourages us to understand the relationship between us, the food we eat, the lifestyle we lead, and how it affects the environment in which we live.

The basic practices include:

- Eat more whole grains, fresh vegetables, and beans.

- Increase the variety of foods consumed.

- Use traditional cooking methods.

- Eat smaller meals more regularly.

- Chew food well to aid digestion.

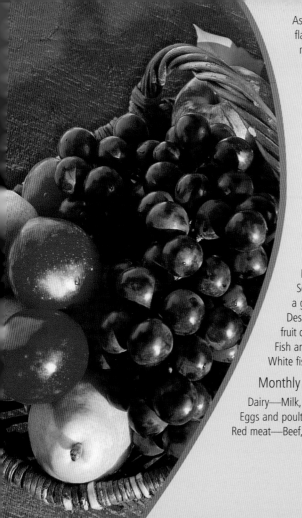

As well as composing meals balanced in flavour, texture, acid and alkali content, macrobiotic eating recommendations are quite different to the traditional nutrition pyramid.

Daily

Whole grains—Brown rice, whole wheat, oats, pasta, bread.
Vegetables and pickles—Balance of leafy, root, cooked, and raw.
Beans and sea vegetables—Lentils, chickpeas, tofu, nori wakame.
Seasonings and condiments—Sea salt, soy sauce, miso.
Vegetable oil.

Weekly

Fruits—Variety of fruits in season.
Seeds and nuts — a good variety.
Desserts—Mostly fruit or grain-based.
Fish and seafood— White fish meat.

Monthly

Dairy—Milk, cheese, yogurt.
Eggs and poultry—Chicken, duck, goose.
Red meat—Beef, lamb, offal.

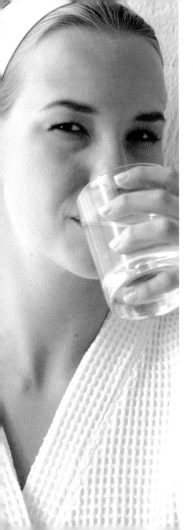

detox diet

There are many different detox programs that you can follow. They can last from 48 hours, to several months.

This is an ideal plan to follow if you need to relax, reduce stress, and rid your body of existing toxins, and reduce the absorption of new toxins by your body. Telltale signs include: feeling sluggish, bloating, recurrent cold or infections, and frequent headaches. While having a break from processing toxins, your liver, kidneys, and digestive system will be able to work more effectively. Your eyes will be brighter, your skin will be clearer, and you will have more vitality and energy.

foods to eat

- Fruit and vegetables.

- Grain, bread, and pasta (wheat/gluten free).

- Pulses, lentils and sprouted beans.

- Cold-pressed oils.

- Nuts and seeds.

- Non-dairy milk.

- Fresh herbs, spices and flavorings.

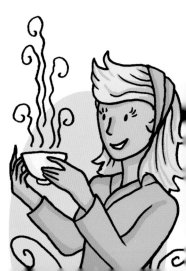

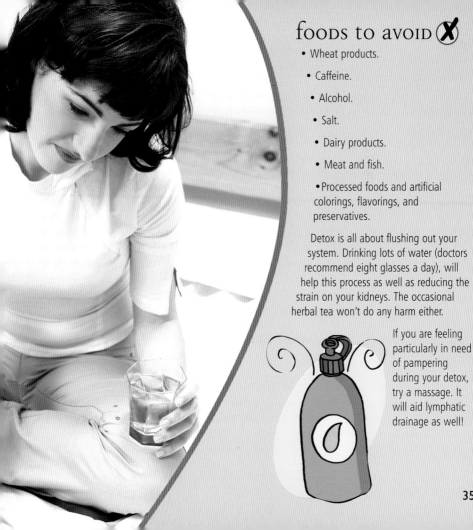

foods to avoid ✗

- Wheat products.
- Caffeine.
- Alcohol.
- Salt.
- Dairy products.
- Meat and fish.
- Processed foods and artificial colorings, flavorings, and preservatives.

Detox is all about flushing out your system. Drinking lots of water (doctors recommend eight glasses a day), will help this process as well as reducing the strain on your kidneys. The occasional herbal tea won't do any harm either.

If you are feeling particularly in need of pampering during your detox, try a massage. It will aid lymphatic drainage as well!

exercise for the body

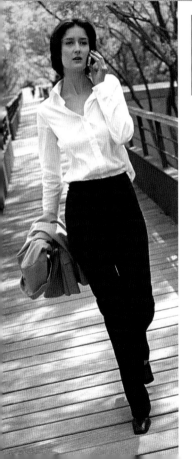

When it comes to exercise and improving cardiovascular fitness, any activity is better than none! It is important to find an activity that is easy for you to do regularly and that you enjoy.

Back to Basics

If you have not done any regular exercise for some time, it is best to start with basic, low-impact exercise and work your way up to more challenging activities. A twenty-minute walk around the block, thirty minutes of housework, or a day gardening, all add up and get you moving. Activity does not need to be organized or continuous, but try to establish a regular pattern.

During your average day these simple changes can make a real difference:

- Park your car a little further away from your destination and walk the extra distance.

- Walk up the stairs instead of taking the elevator.

- Take a break—get up, stretch, and walk around.

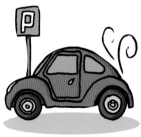

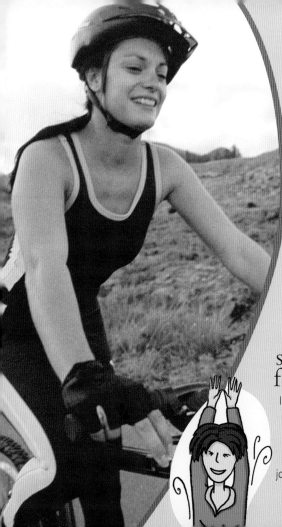

in the groove

When exercise is a part of your life, build regular workouts into your weekly schedule. A routine including at least thirty minutes of cardiovascular activity three or more times a week might include aerobic dancing, brisk walking, jogging, cycling, or swimming. Exercise at an intensity that raises your heart rate to 60-80 percent of your maximum heart rate. (Maximum heart rate = 220 minus your age.)

You can exercise outdoors or in a gym using equipment such as treadmills, bikes, and cross-training machines. Start a sport—it is fun and a great way to make new friends!

Your routine should be enjoyable and comfortable, gradually increasing in intensity and duration.

stretch for flexibility

Inactive muscles become shorter, and their range of motion gets more limited. Reverse that process by doing gentle stretching exercises before and after workouts, and at other times during the week. You could also join a yoga or Pilates class!

37

exercise for the mind

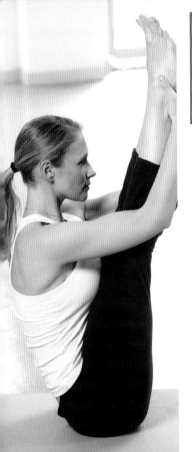

Yoga includes stretching, relaxation, and mind strengthening activities, which are just as important as maintaining tone and cardiovascular fitness. As the body and mind are interconnected and emotions play a big part in determining our health status, built-up stress can have a negative effect on the immune system, and lead to various problems.

Yoga is a very popular therapeutic technique that helps to restore balance and harmony to the mind and body. Through structured poses, you increase flexibility in the joints, stretch, and strengthen muscles, releasing nervous, and physical tension.

thunderbolt or diamond pose

This is a seated posture. Start by sitting back on your heels and placing your knees, legs, and feet together. Keep your back straight and place your hands on top of your thighs, palms down. Breathe gently through your nose. You can hold this position for as long as possible—it is believed to aid digestion.

corpse pose

This is a great pose to start and finish your yoga session. Lie on your back with your legs stretched out together, but not touching, and your arms close to the body, palms facing up. With your eyes closed, and muscles relaxed, concentrate on breathing deeply and slowly. Starting at the top of your head, work your way down to

• *The pictures depict alternative yoga poses.*

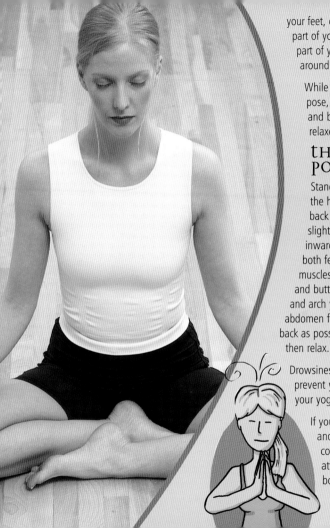

your feet, consciously thinking about each part of your body and then relaxing that part of your body. Hold this pose for around five minutes.

While this may appear to be a simple pose, the purpose of it is for the mind and body to be motionless and relaxed—not as easy as you think!

the mountain posture

Stand with both feet touching from the heel to the big toe. Keep your back straight and arms pressed slightly against the sides, palms facing inward. Balance your weight evenly on both feet, then slightly tighten the muscles in your knees, thighs, stomach, and buttocks. Inhale through the nostrils and arch your back, thrusting the abdomen forward, and tilt the head as far back as possible. Hold while comfortable then relax.

Drowsiness and a restless mind can prevent you from fully benefiting from your yoga session.

If you are sleepy, increase the rate and depth of your breathing. If your concentration wanders, focus your attention on the sensations your body is feeling.

39

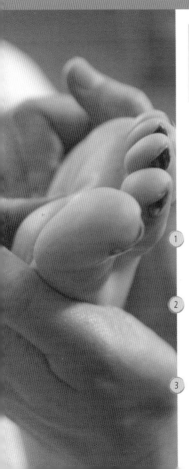

Massage has amazing effects on your health. It improves circulation, relaxes muscles, aids digestion, and, by stimulating the lymph system, speeds up the elimination of toxins and waste products. This promotes a wonderful feeling of well-being.

These simple self-massages can be done at home, or at the office, while watching television, or even on the phone. Use a suitable oil if you are massaging bare skin.

Legs and feet

Follow these steps for a relaxing leg massage. Do one leg first and then start on the other.

1. Starting at the toes, work each foot individually by squeezing firmly and pulling gently. With the thumbs, apply firm pressure down the center of the sole and then either side. Follow this with circular movements on the arch and ball of the foot.

2. Knead the calf muscles of your left leg with both hands, squeezing the muscle away from the bone, then releasing it. Massage your knee, then apply circular pressure with your fingertips around the kneecap. Finish by stroking softly behind your knee up toward your body.

3. Cup your hands around the leg and start by stroking from your ankle, up the calf, over the knee to the top of the thigh. Then with alternate hands, rhythmically knead the thigh by squeezing and releasing the skin. Now smooth your thigh by stroking it from the knee to the top of the thigh, with one hand following the other.

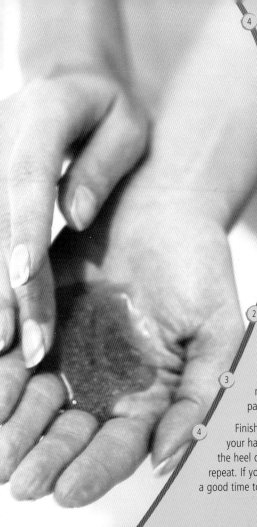

4. Pummel the front and outside of your thighs with loosely clenched fists to help relieve stiffness.

5. To finish, gently soothe from the toes to the thigh, with one hand following the other. Now massage the right leg.

HAND MASSAGE

1. Start by squeezing the hand all over—pressing it between your thumb and fingers. Apply circular pressure over the joints with your thumb. Now hold each finger at its base and pull it gently to stretch it, sliding your grip up the finger and off the tip.

2. Using a finger, stroke between the tendons on the back of the hand, then gently massage the wrist joint.

3. Turn your hand over and apply firm, circular movements with your thumb, working all over the palm and around the wrist.

4. Finish the massage by stroking the palm of your hand from the fingers to the wrist. Push into it with the heel of your other hand, then glide gently back, and repeat. If you end your body massage with your hands, this is a good time to apply a hand lotion to them.

a good night's sleep

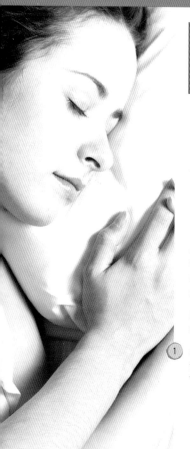

We all have too much to do, and not enough hours to do it in, but we must make sure that "getting things done" does not take over from getting a good night's sleep.

good sleep

Like proper nutrition and exercise, sleep is essential to stay healthy and feel your best. Sleep deprivation, or poor quality of sleep, impacts on both short- and long-term health. It can affect every part of your body and causes loss of mental clarity, fatigue, puffiness and redness of eyes, and loss of facial tone.

How well you sleep at night will directly influence how productive and focused you will be the next day. It is recommended that you try to get around eight hours of sleep every night. However, the quality and quantity of sleep required by each individual to recharge the mind and body will be different.

Here are some suggestions for falling asleep easily and naturally, and for obtaining a more rejuvenating quality of sleep.

1. Give yourself "permission" to go to bed. As hard as it may be to go to bed with things left undone, you need to make sleep a priority. You'll thank yourself in the morning.

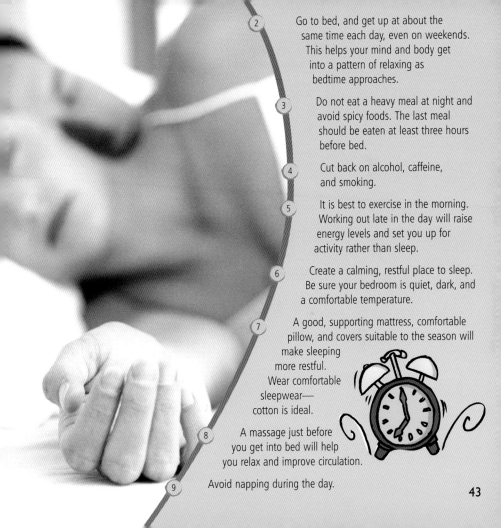

2. Go to bed, and get up at about the same time each day, even on weekends. This helps your mind and body get into a pattern of relaxing as bedtime approaches.

3. Do not eat a heavy meal at night and avoid spicy foods. The last meal should be eaten at least three hours before bed.

4. Cut back on alcohol, caffeine, and smoking.

5. It is best to exercise in the morning. Working out late in the day will raise energy levels and set you up for activity rather than sleep.

6. Create a calming, restful place to sleep. Be sure your bedroom is quiet, dark, and a comfortable temperature.

7. A good, supporting mattress, comfortable pillow, and covers suitable to the season will make sleeping more restful. Wear comfortable sleepwear— cotton is ideal.

8. A massage just before you get into bed will help you relax and improve circulation.

9. Avoid napping during the day.

43

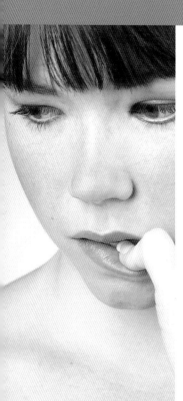

> We all have bad habits but some can have a particularly detrimental effect on your body. Smoking, excessive alcohol, and lack of sleep are just a couple of things that your body will make you regret!

smoking

Although this can be one of the most difficult addictions to break, the benefits to your health and those around you will make it worthwhile. Willpower is driven by your real desire to give up—so you must be mentally prepared. You need to understand why you want to quit—write the reasons down and pin them where you will see them every day. Get professional help! There are lots of government and privately-run organizations that are waiting to help you. So stop making excuses and stop today!

biting finger nails

Biting your nails will not only cause damage to them, but it can also damage your teeth. People often bite their nails out of anxiety, insecurity, to relieve stress, or from force of habit. Biting the tips is not as much of a problem as more aggressive biting that causes the fingers to bleed. Biting or tearing the cuticle can lead to infections and deformed nails.

There are many products available that help to deter biting. Most of these are bitter-tasting liquids applied to the nail.

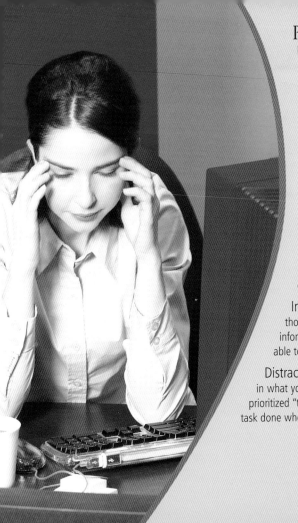

PROCRASTINATION

Not being able to make a decision about something, important or not, can cause a lot of distraction and mental stress. Identifying that you are procrastinating, and then looking at why you are doing so, are the first steps to getting things done.

Unpleasant tasks—Often these are not as bad as you think they are going to be. Get them over with first and then reward yourself for getting them done.

Complex tasks—If something seems insurmountable, break it down into smaller, manageable tasks. Plan and complete it step by step.

Indecision—Take time to get your thoughts together. Gather all of the information or evidence that you need to be able to make an informed decision.

Distraction—Being distracted or not interested in what you have to do is frustrating. Create a prioritized "to-do" list, then allocate time to get the task done when you are at your peak during the day.

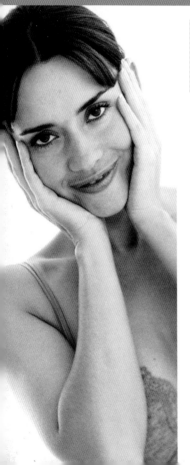

> Unfortunately, it is just a fact of life that sometimes, no matter how well we try to look after ourselves, genes and nature can undo all of our hard work.

pimples and blackheads

Pimples and blackheads are a problem faced by most people, regardless of age. There are many factors that may increase their prevalence, including increased levels of hormones. Your diet also has a huge impact on the overall health of your skin. Drinking more water will help your kidneys flush toxins from your body. Sweat also contains toxins and waste, so have a cleansing shower after exercise. Oil secretion also contributes to blocked pores, so cleansing and toning with products for your skin type will help. Don't pick, squeeze, or scratch pimples or blackheads because oils and germs on your fingers can make them worse! Try the following mask to help with spot break-outs.

bay clay facial mask

4 tablespoons French clay (available in specialist stores or the Internet)
5 dried bay leaves
8½ fl. oz distilled water

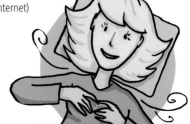

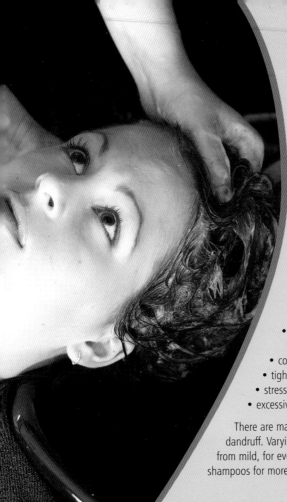

Place the bay leaves into a cup of boiled water and allow to cool. Strain the liquid into a bowl and slowly add it to the clay until it is a fairly thick mixture. Apply to your face, avoiding the eye area, and allow to dry for 15-20 minutes. Rinse with warm water.

DANDRUFF

Some people think dandruff is caused by a lack of cleanliness, but this is far from the truth. Dandruff is a mild inflammation of the scalp causing flaking. These flakes can be extremely noticeable on the hair, and frequently fall on the shoulder, making the problem highly visible. Dandruff is often seasonal, being most severe during winter and milder during the summer. It can be caused by many factors including:

- excessive use of sprays, gels, and other hair products;
- cold weather and drying indoor heating;
- tight-fitting hats and scarves;
- stress, anxiety, and tension; and
- excessive use of hair dryers and curlers.

There are many treatments available to help control dandruff. Varying in strength and ingredients, these range from mild, for everyday use, to stronger, medicated shampoos for more persistent dandruff.

47

CONCLUSION

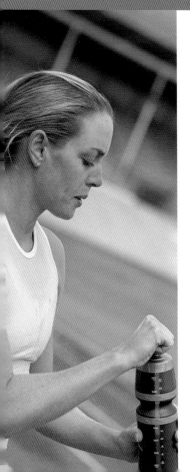

putting it all together

Remembering that all parts of our bodies are linked in some way reminds us how easily the good and bad things that we do can have an impact on our health. Remember, you don't just drink water because you are thirsty—it also ensures your organs function properly and keeps skin, hair, nails, and many other parts of your body hydrated.

Taking time out to care for your mind and body can be very satisfying. It will give you a chance to draw breath, refocus and remember what you really love in life. You should never feel guilty for thinking about yourself once in a while.

try it at home

There are lots of ideas in this book that you can try at home—but how about really treating yourself and going to a salon or beauty parlor? A whole body mud wrap, full-body massage, or just a manicure and pedicure can make you feel really great!

Picture Credits
Imagesource; pages 2, 6, 13, 17-19, 23, 28, 29, 40, 41
Photos.com; pages 4, 5, 7,8, 9-12, 14-16, 20-22, 30, 31, 34, 36, 37, 43, 45-48
Ablestock; pages 24, 27, 32, 33, 35, 38, 39, 42, 44

Remember, the topics in this book are just recommendations and it is advised that you should check with your doctor, dermatologist, or other physician before trying new products or making dramatic changes to your lifestyle.